DRY FAST

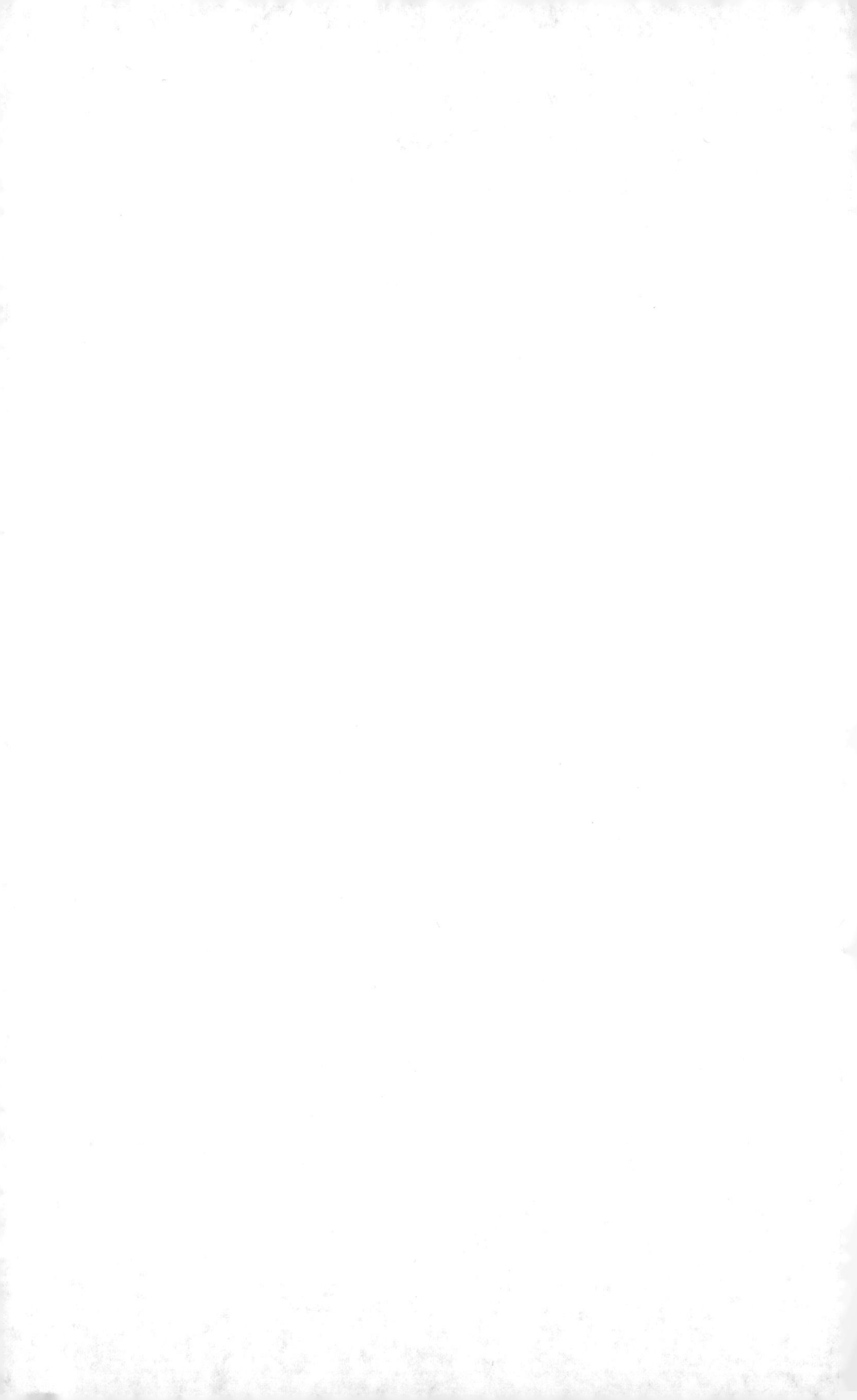

CONTENTS

CHAPTER 1

CHAPTER 2

CHAPTER 3

CHAPTER 4

CHAPTER 5

CHAPTER 6

i)   Dry fasting in preparation for rapture ground

ii)   Dry fasting for long life

iii) The pros and cons

iv) Clearing the misconceptions (hearsay) about dry fasting

v)   Advantages of dry fasting over the other types of fasting

vi) Super benefits of dry fasting.

vii)   What to do during the process of dry fasting

CHAPTER 7

i)   How to break dry fast safely

ii)   The rules to be observed strictly (1-7)

iii) My own experience

iv) Fasting helps in persecution.

CONCLUSION

INTRODUCTION.

The most effective tool in the hands of every person on earth today is the most ignored and resisted .Fasting is the most powerful thing in nature to allow for self healing without side effects . The body of a human is a pharmacy on it's own .If only given enough time it will heal itself . Every disease under the earth can be cured through fasting only if done early enough .

Fasting is not only for curing but it is effective in sychronising the eight dimensions of a human being.Your whole being gets in harmony .You get physically fit .Intellectually you get mental clarity and very vivid memory -no brain fogs .
Emotional healing and stability is one of the benefits that comes automatically as long as you fast.Socially you become more intuitive .This further helps you to identify and keep the toxic friends away from you .Since your emotions are healed during the process of dry fast .Moving along with people becomes very easy .
Spiritual dimension -it is like during dry fast and especially the prolonged one your spirit becomes alive and very active . Many who go for a prolonged dry fast become aware of this abilities .They get to level where the spirit world becomes so real to them .Spirit do not eat and that is why when you stop to eat it easy for you to have a commune within and without.

Vocational dimension ,those who do dry fast become very effective in their work .They become the best of the employees and if they are into their own businesses they get more creative and independent.They also get very new ideas becomes their minds are very clear .They do become enterpreneurs and live in finacial freedom . Money is never an issue with those who practice frequent fasts .Those who live a lifestyle of fasting have all they need .Most often they do not eat ,they also lose ambitious motives -they move in a very free calm spirit .This are people very close to the nature .They do not harm fellow humans nor the environment . Actually dry fast is best done in clean environment in the nature where birds chirps ,no industries ,no electronics ,no pollutions .

CHAPTER 1

WHAT IS DRY FAST

There are two kinds of Dry Fast to start with.
a) Hard
b) Soft

Fasting without consuming anything including water .

What is a Hard Dry Fast?

This is the Hebrew fast, the Absolute fast or total fast or true fast.

This is done with total elimination of water. The one practising this fasting does not allow contact with water.No water touching the body that means:

No washing dishes, (Wear gloves)

No taking baths or shower (very important)

No brushing teeth

No washing face or hands or legs

No drinking juice or water

No eating any food-nothing from outside goes down the gut.

However with soft dry fast, the one fasting can allow the body to contact water but not drink. Meaning you can bath, brush your teeth and wash face.

During this kind of fasting one cuts off the world,no television,no phones,no newspapers,no visits.Totally secluded from the world.

You switch off television, radio, phones and anything that connects you to the world.

You switch on to worship. Prayer and study of the word of God. Listening more to the Holy Spirit, try to be spiritually alert.To be able to hear from God.Connect with your innerself or inner-man .

Create a notebook for recording your experiences which include physical, psychological and spiritual changes.

Dry fasting is the most effective in healing; it brings about emotional, psychological as well as physical healing.Dry fast will change you to be another man .The super you will be unleashed .The faith in you will be real .The faith that cannot be defeated by anything .

THE BACKGROUND

From a religious perspective. It is the fast that Moses,Elijah ,Esther,David,Jesus,disciples practised.
It is the fast of the Bible

It was and still is used for repentance during the day of Atonement everyone in the nation of Israel fast from sunset to sunset about 25hrs once every year during Yom Kippur.

Leviticus 16:29-31

And this shall be a statute for ever
unto you: that in the seventh month,
on the tenth day of the month, ye
shall afflict your souls, and do no work
at all, whether it be one of your own
country, or a stranger that sojourneth
among you: For on that day shall
the priest make an atonement for
you, to cleanse you, that ye may

*be clean from all your sins before
the LORD.   It shall be a sabbath
of rest unto you, and ye shall afflict
your souls, by a statute for ever.*

This shall be a statute forever for you.

*In the seventh month, on the tenth day
of the month, you shall afflict your
souls and do no work at all, whether
a native of your own country or a
stranger who dwells among you.*

*"For on that day the priest shall
make atonement for you, to cleanse
you, that you may be clean from
all your sins before the Lord.*

*It is a Sabbath of solemn rest
for you and you shall afflict your
souls, It is a statute forever.*

During Yom Kippur the Jews do a dry fast and also do not Work and do not wear shoes. They abstain from sex, they do not wash. This is the pattern we are to emulate .With the help of the Holy Spirit we can do better .Through the blood of Jesus we are more than conquerors .

It is not only during the repentance that a fast is done in the Bible but also when one prepares to take a sacred meal.

When one wants to have visions from heaven.When you fast your dreams become very clear . Anything you ask God respond instantly .Y ou will be able to operate in the prophetic with ease and accuracy . As long as you are baptised in the Holy Spirit ,the spiritual gifts will operate with ease in your life .Joel 2:28 .

When one needs the fruit of the womb especially to have strength to be able to bear children.Cases of infertility .

Ex 23:26. There shall nothing cast their young, nor be barren, in thy land: the number of thy days I will fulfil.

 When one responds to a serious spiritual need – this is clearly demonstrated in the life of David

2 Sam 12:16. David therefore besought God for the child; and David fasted, and went in, and lay all night upon the earth.

When mourning the death of king Saul and his children.

1 Sam 31:13. 13 *And they took their bones, and buried them under a tree at Jabesh, and fasted seven days. They took their bones and buried them under the tamarisk tree at Jabesh and fasted Seven days.*

The authority to proclaim a public fast was rested in the elders of local community in Israel.

1 Kings 21:8-128 So she wrote letters in Ahab's name, and sealed them with his seal, and sent the letters unto the elders and to the nobles that were in his city, dwelling with Naboth. 9 And she wrote in the letters, saying, Proclaim a fast, and set Naboth on high among the people: 10 And set two men, sons of Belial, before him, to bear witness against him, saying, Thou didst blaspheme God and the king. And then carry him out, and stone him, that he may die. 11 And the men of his city, even the elders and the nobles who were the inhabitants in his city, did as Jezebel had sent unto them, and as it was written in the letters which she had sent unto them. 12 They proclaimed a fast, and set Naboth on high among the people.

clothing *was* sackcloth: I humbled my soul with fasting; and my prayer returned into mine own bosom Fasting is done to win divine forgiveness. Psalm 35:13 But as for me, when they were sick, my therefore fasting is an expression of remorse, submission and getting out of the way for God to take pre-eminence. It allows deep fellowship with God as did Moses and Elijah. It allows vision as experienced by Daniel . It was used by queen Esther to avert genocide. Evil plans of Haman. Yes ,it can be used even today to avert any calamity .

It was used to seek God's direct intervention during war time.

 Judges 20:26, Then all the children of Israel, and all the people, went up, and came unto the house of God, and wept, and sat there before the LORD, and fasted that day until even, and offered burnt offerings and peace offerings before the LORD.

1Chronicle 20:3 And he brought out the people that *were* in it, and cut *them* with saws, and with harrows of iron, and with axes. Even so dealt David with all the cities of the children of Ammon. And David and all the people returned to Jerusalem.

1 Sam 7:6 And they gathered together to Mizpeh, and drew water, and poured *it* out before the LORD, and fasted on that day, and said there, We have sinned against the LORD. And Samuel judged the children of Israel in Mizpeh.

It was used to avert the threat of divine punishment.

Jonah 3:5 So the people of Nineveh believed God, and proclaimed a fast, and put on sackcloth, from the greatest of them even to the least of them.Fasting is accomplished by

a) Prayer
   Judges 20:26Then all the children of Israel, and all the people, went up, and came unto the house of God, and wept, and sat there before the LORD, and fasted that day until even, and offered burnt offerings and peace offerings before the LORD.

Before you fast

You need to write your prayer points ,make a list of your

needs. Your requests write them down link a promise from Gods words to the prayer request.Get from the promises of God what is aligned to your need.

Example: For strength Deut 33:25Thy shoes *shall be* iron and brass; and as thy days, *so shall* thy strength *be.*

Healing **1 Peter 2:24Who his own self bare our sins in his own body on the tree, that we, being dead to sins, should live unto righteousness: by whose stripes ye were healed.**

For Fruit of the womb **Deut 28:5 Blessed shall be thy basket and thy store.**

Power to break curses Gal 3:13Christ hath redeemed us from the curse of the law, being made a curse for us: for it is written, Cursed is every one that hangeth on a tree

Power over demonic oppression **Luke 10:19 Behold, I give unto you power to tread on serpents and scorpions, and over all the power of the enemy: and nothing shall by any means hurt you.**

Remember to always say out loud the scriptures and repeatedly during the fast.What you want to see confess,declare.If it is healing declare ,am healed.

Repeatedly quote the verse that corresponds to your need during the fast. Do it as many times as possible (through the fasting period). Speak the word all the time.It is the secret of the flow of the anointing,you attract the anointing based on the word you read,meditate,believe and speak .Jesus had done it when on the cross -He paid it all . You only need to claim the promises . Fasting is only helping you to get out of the way so that you can contact that power of the anointing but the real work had been finished on the cross.

When you pray, meditate, walk, sleep and stand – use the word,the name of Jesus and the blood . Remember also to keep praising not complaining.Ther e is power in praise .Prayer should be 99% praise .

Use the word as a sword in your mouth not hand – This is the way to claim the promises and defeat the enemy.Declare the word .

Rev. 19:15 And out of his mouth goeth a sharp sword, that with it he should smite the nations: and he shall rule them with a rod of iron: and he treadeth the winepress of the fierceness and wrath of Almighty God

Fasting is accomplished by

Giving Sacrifice to God **1 Sam 7 : 6** And they gathered together to Mizpeh, and drew water, and poured *it* out before the LORD, and fasted on that day, and said there, We have sinned against the LORD. And Samuel judged the children of Israel in Mizpeh

Giving offering

Giving to God through giving to the needy /poor **Prov 19:17** He that hath pity upon the poor lendeth unto the LORD; and that which he hath given will he pay him again.

Pay your tithe **Matt 23:23** Woe unto you, scribes and Pharisees, hypocrites! for ye pay tithe of mint and anise and cummin, and have omitted the weightier *matters* of the law, judgment, mercy, and faith: these ought ye to have done, and not to leave the other undone.

Heb 7:8 *And here men that die receive tithes; but there he receiveth them, of whom it is witnessed that he liveth.*

During the period of fasting, it is time to reflect to determine where you went wrong and it is also time to search the

scriptures for answers to the reason for
the fast. Never fast without a reason.

It is time to investigate self in order to determine the course of your life. Where are you taking your destiny?
Where are you taking the destiny of your life/family?
Where are you taking the destiny of your ministry?
It is time to ask God . It is also time to listen to the Holy Spirit. It is time to turn away from your own ways and thoughts. Your own thoughts and plans must now submit to God's will.
It is time for God's will to be done only God's way matter.
It is time to crucify the flesh. It is time to yield to the Holy Spirit and follow his lead.

CHAPTER 2

PREPARATION BEFORE THE FAST

First things first.
A man can endure all, knowing why or for what he is doing .
Matt 24:13 *But he that shall endure unto the end, the same shall be saved.*

Prepare Psychologically;

Prepare self, mentally for the fact that you are going to experience temporary "pain" for permanent gain.
Focus on the results and what you will gain if you faithfully complete your fast.
During the fast our body is very happy but our subconscious mind is not . It is actually where the real battle is taking place.

So when your mind tells you to eat tell it " I do not want to eat'
Fear is only a result of less understanding on the adventure we undertake.
Remember the power of motivation. Before starting the fast answer the question
For What?
What do I want to achieve?
How much do I really need it?Why must the answer only come through a fast?What happens to my situation if I don't take any action?

NUTRITION PREPARATION

Prepare in advance two to three months before the dry fast.
Start to eat the right food. Take eleminate junk food from your diet .
It will surprise you the types of food to totally avoid.
i)   Meat (beef, pork, lamb)
ii)   Coffee
iii)   Canned food (food in tins)
iv)   No smoking
v)   No alcoholic drinks

You are allowed to switch on to in your menu:
White meat-for those not in strict vegeterian diet; fish, poultry, dairy products, honey
Cooked vegetables
Drinks clean filtered water, mineral water , herbal tea

While I was still new with dry fast ,I took coffee and tried to fast .I could not go past 48 hours because I was shaking as if all my muscles and the entire body was lacking energy .I kept trying for about three times but I could not .I later realized it was coffee and from that time I stopped taking coffee . Coffee and dry fast do not go hand in hand .You must just remove coffee totally the same way I did .

CLEANING THE INTESTINAL

This process of cleaning include the liver ,blood ,small intestine and the large intestine .

Preparation for Dry fast:

If you are under medication especially if you depend on medicine ,you need to take activated charcoal for four days .Thirty minutes before every meal . It is very effective in draining all toxic things in your system.It is always used to help neutralise poison . Since it is negative it takes everything positive.Should not be taken consecutivelly for more than five days .It clears every positive charge in the body.

After the forth day you wait until the next day and take castor oil commensurate to your weight .For example if you weigh 70kgs then take 70ml per the major meal times for only two days . This will also help you in flushing the activated charcoal from your system .

Alternativelly for flushing your system you can do salt flush .
It is a highly effective way to remove wastes that are stuck on your gut especially the large intestine . It expels toxins and waste. I have successfully done it several times .Putting salt in your body may not be good for evryone .

How to perform a salt flush.One table spoon on one litre of fresh water drink shortest time possible the first thing in the morning. If you want to perform it the perfect way .Use seven full tablespoon salt in seven litres .Drink within seven hours as you perform shank prakshalana exercise .Check this on our YouTube channel-Dry Fast .

After a salt flush you will have
i) Better digestion
ii) Increased energy
iii) You will feel fresh
iv) And even loss some weight

Preparation for Dry Fast.

Liver Cleaning

It is very important to clean your liver before undertaking the course of a dry fast. For a period of at least one week.
Required to be taken
Lemon Fruits, Carrots apples olive oil;.
Leafy Green Vegetables,celery and pears .
Garlic
Off course plenty of sleep.

Now that you have prepared you need to know how to start.
You can do a three day Juice fast then break, eat normally
Then do a three day water fast then break, eat normally for three days.
Then you can start the dry fast. Fasting can take 24 hrs
Two days
Three Days
Four Days
Five Days then break then with 2 litres of warm water.
You rest for three days or more then you can start again. Do as your will and your strength takes you. But remember this is just the beginning of the journey it is not final. Fasting should be a

lifestyle.

Carry out detoxicification depending on your health status.

DO NOT DISCUSS WITH ANYONE NEITHER FOR OR AGAINST THE FAST.

Matt 6:16 *Moreover when ye fast, be not, as the hypocrites, of a sad countenance: for they disfigure their faces, that they may appear unto men to fast. Verily I say unto you, They have their reward*

CHAPTER 3

Types of Fasting

Complete Dry fast.
Anthing beyond five days and nights is a long dry fast.
This takes either 5,7, 9,10 , 11 or 12 days .

It helps to get rid of different diseases especially the serious ones. It is helps to unleash the hidden reserves of creativity intelligence and leads to discoveries.You become mentally sharp.Your mental clarity goes on top of the roof.

It cleanses the body therefore allows maintenance of health, give rest to all organs of the gastrointestinal tract, stimulates creative activity of man, raises emotional and imaginative perception of the outside world.

It strengthens a person's will and faith.

It also helps in reducing excessive weight since averagely per day one loses one kilogram.

During this kind of fast the pores on the skin open and takes water into the body in form of moisture. This is the reason it must be done in a very clean environment.

It normalizes blood pressure, as well as the activities of nervous system.

It can be done at home under the right condition or in fasting centers, as long as the place is environmentally clean.Someone in a clean environment.

It allows healing of infectious diseases e.g acute viral hepatitis (cancer- adenomas prostate) : Uterine cancer, severe somatic diseases(asthma, hereditary- degenerative nervous system diseases, coronary heart diseases.

Inflammatory diseases (prostatis, myocarditis) e.t.c.

This method of fasting allows the second acidosis crisis to be reached and passed. After passing it one reaches ten or eleven days. One get to concentrate on the important issues of healing.

This method of fasting must be held out door, in clean environment.

2. The Interminent Fasting

Three methods of interminent fast are:

i.alternate day fasting

ii.periodic fasting

iii.daily time restricted feeding.

You always choose what your body can manage.You listen to your body.

This is done one day drinking and eating,

two days, fasting two days eating and drinking

Three days dry fasting, three days eating and drinking.

Four days dry fasting, four days eating and drinking

Five days fast then the faster rests for at least a month (30) days or at most 3 months then starts again.

   a) 1-1

   b) 2-2

   c).3-3

   d) 4-4

   e).5-5

This is the easiest way to fast. It has no risks involved. One can do it at home safely without supervision. Only remember the rules of breaking the fast as long as it has passed two days. You must break with water first (2litres) then you can start to drink the blended juices

,yoghurt etc You always treat your stomach as that of a new born baby.Avoid processed food by all means.Do not break your fast with solid food.Just use the liquids .

FRACTIONAL DRY FASTING (DIVIDED)

This also another way of dry fasting but it more vigorous.

This way of fast you do divide the days and fast in series.Divide the number of days you want to fast. It is done in phases. It aims at reaching both acidotic crisis, which is the first and the second.

The one fasting breaks the first phase of fast after reaching acidotic crisis which takes place between the third day to the seventh. Then the fasters rests for three days to maximum of two months taking a lot of fluids and natural juices .

 You break the fast normally -observing the rules of breaking the dry fasting.

Then the person fasts for 9 , 10 , 11 or maximum 12 days.

 I mean day and night . Not eating in the evening or any other time .During dry fast you do not consume anything .Your body will be taking water from the air and there will be endogenous feeding,the body feeds from within from the fat reserves ,weak cells,bacteria within the gut .

   a) 7- 10-11   b) 5-10-9   c) 6-10-10

What is most important is passing the acidiotic crisis which when it happens you feel as if fire is burning you in your blood or the whole body . Then you can rest between five to 10 days and do the third and final phase of the fast which must not last longer than seven days.

 The numbers in red are the fasting days while the black are the resting days -rehydration and consuming only raw foods to allow the body heal .During the time of resting you hydrate properly. You have to not return to normal eating of junk food.You can choose what consume but it is highly recommended that if you are fasting for healing you switch to raw food, natural juices and plenty of water then you can resume your fast.Fasting is a natural thing that should not scare you.It is actually to your greatest benefit.You cannot compare fasting with any method of healing. Wild animals listen to there intuitons and do fasting naturally without supervision.You only need to gather all the neccessary information to start.The experienced fasters will tell you they had some fear before starting but after experimenting they found it easier and very beneficial.It is the easiest and with greatest re- sults -dry fast .

Little is known about dry fast,because juice and water fast are the most popular since many have information on them.The guide- lines and rules of dry fast are to be strictly followed.The good thing with dry fast is that when you want to start coming back to normal feeding it is quite easy ,as long as you have followed the strict guidelines of breaking the dry fast.

I do break the fast with warm water alone and then later put a lit- tle natural lemon juice from lemon fruits.One or two are enough for me .

Prolonged Dry Fast Days.
The rehydration period should be between ten days to to two months before you continue the fast .During the rehydration strictly use raw food , juices and fluids .Fluids can be vegetable soups etc .Do not eat beef or procossed food like soda because you are still in the process of the fast and healing is made easier that way .

For power of the Holy Spirit or any other reason of fasting -avoid interrupting your fast . Do not interrupt by introducing solids be- cause even your intestines or digestive system is not ready . Just apply patience but feast on the juices like beetroot,watermelon etc .

There is another method of dry fast that goes beyond 12 days and it is used by those who have very long experience with dry fast .This method is developed over a long period of time . Someone starts with nutrition ,where you totally turn to vegan and eat nuts . You come out from cooked food .Eating raw for a long period of time until the body transition totally .

The fast is then done in increasing cirlce eg if you did 3 days and nights next time you aim at 5 days and nights .
If you did 12 days next time you do 15 days and nights .If you did 20 next time you do 25 ,you keep growing the circle until you reach 40 days or more . Sat Marga who I was priviledged to interview on our YouTube channel called Dry Fast did upto 50 days and nights .

.

The fourth way of a dry fasting is soft dry fast.

Where one does not eat or drink but allows full contact with water.
In bathing taking showers rinsing the mouth washing the face, swimming etc .During the fast you have contact with water but you do not drink it.
This can last up to even 18 or 21 days but it is not the Hebrew fast.
It is not the biblical fast and the skin which has over 96 million pores takes water fully.
This type of fast won't give the faster the same results as total dry fast.

THE FIFTH :COMBINED TYPE OF DRY FASTING

Combined water and dry fast
You fast between 2 to 3 days and then take water for 24 hours then again 2-3 days for 30days or even forty days.The safe way to dry fast for a long time .During the rehydration you can also

take juices.With this kind you can reach four days with ease and safely.If you are fasting for the power of God to pass through and touch and change the life of others by them getting their needs met ,it is the best.It is better than full juice fast or water fast.The [power that works within you will be released so mighty until yourself you get shocked.

You are still on the fasting mode even when you take only water or juice.If you are a minister of the gospel this is highly recom-mended.If you just seeking God for other needs different from healing this is recommended to you too.Why do we always fast .It is not to get the power because the power is already within us as Holy Spirit filled believers.We fast because we want to allow the power within us to pass through us and change the lives of the other people.We fast to have the power of the HolySpirit operate . The flesh has to give way for the HolySpirit to take 100% control .

In Africa and the rest of the world you must have the anointing of breaking curses ,casting out demons,healing too is a must.The needs of people is great.We have to come out of our hiding and go with Jesus for souls .

You can also do two or three days and night fasts and then break with water and juices within a period of two hours and continue with the fast again for two or three days . Keep going this will take you to 14 or 21 or 28 or 30 or even forty days and nights Itt all depend with what you need and how you need it . It is also worth noticing that for you to gain full benefits of the fast your mind must be in the fast .You do not stuggle or have battle in the mind why you are not eating while others are .You must be at peace with what your doing to gain a hundred percent benefits . List the things you need to see as the results after the fast . See the benefits of fasting and know that it is not you to be pitied because you de-nied yourself food but those who are eating the way to the grave . Those who do not fast are to be pitied ,they are headed to a very tough times ahead . If you deny yourself food you are one of the most priviledged people on the face of the planet .

What you eat after the fast is very crucial . Go greens and exercise .Have a wonderful mental health .Rejoice always .

CHAPTER4

FACTS ON DRY FAST

The body is put under stringent (tough) condition hence it has to produce both nutrients and water.

Tissues of the body are split more quickly in a short time. One day fast is equal to 3 days on water.

During water fast, water from outside enters the body but during dry fasting each cell in the absence of water from outside produces it own water by burning toxins, weak and dying cells. Each cell turns into a mini furnace reactor that is thermo-nuclear reactions happens under such condition only the strongest and best cells survives.

The cells that survive must be very healthy. The water that is produced from the body is of very high quality. The old water is replaced with healthy super living water.

During dry fasting one will not feel hunger as when undertaking water fast.

If the body does not take in dead heavy water, it means the blood is not getting many harmful substance e therefore the blood has time to filter harmful elements this makes the blood plasma to become as transparent as glass rather as clear as crystal. Everything comes in harmony, including

CLOTTING FACTOR

Dry fasting cleans the blood more completely, than by dialysis or hardware blood purification. Consequently all process in the body associated with blood will be performed almost perfect.

Any swelling in the body disappears. Dry fasting works as anti inflammation, No swelling can happen without water. Deficit of water is extremely damaging to the inflammation.

Healthy strong cells receive additional energy and water, and the sick the viruses and bacteria cannot.

Bacteria viruses, worms without water perish instantly.

During dry fasting because of absence of water from outside the body the cell turns into their own furnace fusion reaction.

Each cell turns into a mini reactor. This allows for an increase in internal temperature of the body. Though this increase in temperature cannot be registered on a thermometer, it is felt by people during the dry fast as an inner glow, fire or chills.

This destroys very poison slag even cancer cells.

It also speeds up the recovery period with increase in temperature - it becomes easier for the immune system to track down and kill all foreigners.

Dry Fast helps in weight loss

Since the fat tissue consist of 90% water and it is this water that is produced during the dry fast.

During dry fasting adipose tissue burns in exactly 3 times faster than during fasting with water.

It splits deposits of fats and then is no recovery or restoration of the same after the fast.

It does not cost anything and most importantly it is harmless.

During the fasting organism takes from the reserves only what is important/ necessary at the moment and not something that is artificially imposed from the outside.

Dry Fast has renewing effect

The weak disease and degenerated cells cannot stand extreme

conditions. They die and decompose leaving only the strong, working and stable cells

Fasting helps to eliminate worthless, weak, sick and harmful cells.

This can be called cell parasites because they do not perform their functions work responsibly. It is much better if we get rid of them not allowing them to die natural death.

When they are left before they die, they manage to create for themselves similar offspring dead and broken wreck(like father like son)

Therefore the cells that survive after dry fast create strong and high quality offspring during cell multiplication.

DRY FASTING FOR HEALING

The following diseases disappear during dry fasting
    1. Infertility
Ovarian cyst, mastopathy, myoma , uterine fibroids, uterine polyps, endometriosis, inflammation in the pelvis.

    2. Disease of musculoskeletal system.
Rheumatoid arthritis, osteoarthritis deformans, anklylosing spondylitis, infections polyarthritis.
    3. Bronchopulmonary diseases.
Bronchial asthma
Obstructive bronchitis
Pulmonary sarcoidosis
    4. Diseases of the the cardiovascular system
Hypertension diseases stage i or ii
Neurocirculatory dystonia of hypertensive type:
Atheroscelerosis of celebral vessels

    5. Neurological diseases
Osteochondrosis
Protusion and herniated disc
Spinal headache.
Neuralgia, Lumbago, sciatica
    6. Diseases of gastrointestinal track:
Chronic gastritis and gastroduodenitis, Chronic enteristis and colitis. Biliary dyskinesia, syndrome irritable
    7. Skin diseases
Atopic dermatitis
Chronic urticaria
Eczema psoriasis
Trophic ulcers
    8. Urological diseases
Chronic pyelonephritis,
Cystitis, prostatitis

Prostate adenoma

THOSE NOT PERMITTED
TO USE DRY FAST

It is very important to notice that fasting can heal all diseases but it must be started early before the disease has advanced.It is therefore recommended you do practice a weekly fast once for 24 hours.Monthly fast between three to five days.After every four months or changing season fast 5 to seven days and nights . Annually do a 9,10 ,11 or 12 days once .This will put you your body immunity in a state it cannot get sick -prevention is better than cure .Do not wait until you are sick ,very sick to turn to dry fast as the last .

Those who are suffering from the following diseases in there advanced state are not allowed to dry fast.

Believe God for healing-have faith .All things are possible to him that believes .With God nothing is impossible.

Malignant tumors
Hematological malignancies
Active tuberculosis of the lungs and other organs
Hyperthyroidism and other endocrine diseases
Cirrhosis of the liver
Pyo – inflammatory diseases of the respiratory and abdominal cavity.
Circulatory failure ii and iii degrees persistent irregular heart rhythm and conductions.
Pronounced underweight
Thrombophlebitis and thrombosis
Note
Expectant mothers (during pregnancy)   and lactating

mothers (those who are breastfeeding.
Children
Those who are under 14 years
Old men and women of 70 years and above .

These must be adhered to failure to take care of the warning and risks you take the full responsibility .

Though expectant mothers can take activated charcoal for four days maximum then fast only on water for five days .Warning, fasting past five days causes abortion .

CHAPTER5

DRY FASTING TO CHANGE BAD HABITS

You have so struggled with some bad habits what we call continuous circle in sin.

You fall and wake up then only fall again over and over the same sin.

This could be sexual sin, alcoholism, outburst of wrath, Jealousy, smoking, hatred, taking offence, holding grudges over the years until you are not even sure whether it is sin.

Even love of pleasure, love of money, lying, drunkardness, prostitution, on and on ....

Dry fast has power to change a person totally from inside out within and without.

Anything called sin – disobedience can be confessed and repented off but how to totally have dominion over the works of the flesh is to work in the spirit.

Dry fasting creates the platform to totally deliver you from sin and switches you on into the spirit as long as you are a child of God.

This is the secret of how to live free from all sins as mentioned in the bible without holiness no one will see God.

Hebrews 12:14 *Follow peace with all men, and holiness, without which no man shall see the Lord:*
It is important to note that three days dry fast is used for repentance just as the Ninevites did, but if any anyone wants to see a total change from bad habits it is necessary to go beyond seven days continuously day and night.
Nine or ten days are highly recommended for very strong habits that may as well have formed your personality.
Example
smoking
Evil imaginations, evil thought
Laziness
Pornography
Doubt
Corruption
Depression, self pity, stress
Unbelief
Envy, jealousy , covetousness
Sexual sin (adultery, fornication, bestiality (having sex with animals), homosexuality, having sex with the dead or spirits or snakes or spiritual husbands.
False gifts of the Holy Spirit
False Prophesies, faking miracles, condemnation, apostasy, presumptuousness, hatred, strive., seducing spirits, spirit of heaviness, All drug addictions, Robbery, Blindness, Confusion, Gossip, cursing, fear, Blasphemy, Spirit of death, self willed temptation, inferiority, occult, negative confessions, mockery, hypnosis, medicine, dependency, poverty, all forms of strongholds e.t.c.
Dry fasting is a way of putting yourself away so that God can have His way for you and yours (family, job, ministry, and nation)
Combined with prayers and relevant scriptures it gives all the results prayer can offer in hundreds fold – return .
1.Victorious Triumph 2 Chronicle 20:22-*23And when they*

began to sing and to praise, the LORD set ambushments against the children of Ammon, Moab, and mount Seir, which were come against Judah; and they were smitten.   23 For the children of Ammon and Moab stood up against the inhabitants of mount Seir, utterly to slay and destroy them: and when they had made an end of the inhabitants of Seir, every one helped to destroy another.

2.Blessings Gen 12;2-3 *And I will make of thee a great nation, and I will bless thee, and make thy name great; and thou shalt be a blessing: 3 And I will bless them that bless thee, and curse him that curseth thee: and in thee shall all families of the earth be blessed.*

3.Healing Deut 7:*15 And the LORD will take away from thee all sickness, and will put none of the evil diseases of Egypt, which thou knowest, upon thee; but will lay them upon all them that hate thee.*

4.Deliverance Mark 16:17 *And these signs shall follow them that believe; In my name shall they cast out devils; they shall speak with new tongues;*

5.Peace John 14:27 *Peace I leave with you, my peace I give unto you: not as the world giveth, give I unto you. Let not your heart be troubled, neither let it be afraid*

6.Joy Neh 8: 10 *Peace I leave with you, my peace I give unto you: not as the world giveth, give I unto you. Let not your heart be troubled, neither let it be afraid*

7.Love 1 Cor 13:13 *Peace I leave with you, my peace I give unto you: not as the world giveth, give I unto you. Let not your heart be troubled, neither let it be afraid*

8.Success 1 Kings 2:13 *Peace I leave with you, my peace I give unto you: not as the world giveth, give I unto you. Let not your heart be troubled, neither let it be afraid,* Joshua 1:5-9 *There shall not any man be able to stand before thee all the days of thy life: as I was with Moses, so I will be with thee: I will not fail thee, nor forsake thee. 6 Be strong and of a good courage: for unto this people shalt thou divide for an inheritance the land, which I sware unto their fathers to give them. 7 Only be thou strong and very courageous, that thou mayest observe to do according to all the law, which Moses my servant commanded thee: turn not from it to the right hand or to the left, that thou mayest prosper whithersoever thou goest. 8 This book of the law shall not depart out of thy mouth; but thou shalt meditate therein day and night, that thou mayest observe to do according to all that is written therein: for then thou shalt make thy way prosperous, and then thou shalt have good success. 9 Have not I commanded thee? Be strong and of a good courage; be not afraid, neither be thou dismayed: for the LORD thy God is with thee whithersoever thou goest*

9.Wisdom James 1:5*If any of you lack wisdom, let him ask of God, that giveth to all men liberally, and upbraideth not; and it shall be given him.*

Knowledge Hosea 4:6 *My people are destroyed for lack of knowledge: because thou hast rejected knowledge, I will also reject thee, that thou shalt be no priest to me: seeing thou hast forgotten the law of thy God, I will also forget thy children.*

10.Power to have heavenly vision

11.To hear from God directly and clearly

12.To understand the secrets in the scriptures (revelations) Luke 24:31-*32And their eyes were opened, and they knew him; and he vanished out of their sight. 32 And they said one to another, Did not our heart burn within us, while he talked with us by the way, and while he opened to us the scriptures?*

13.To have Miracles

14.Power to win souls effectively Acts2:41: *Then they that gladly received his word were baptized: and the same day there were added unto them about three thousand souls.*

Supernatural Church growth Acts 13: 44*But when they departed from Perga, they came to Antioch in Pisidia, and went into the synagogue on the sabbath day, and sat down.*

DRY FASTING FOR ANOINTING

The only source of the anointing is the Holy spirit.When you fast and pray you allow the Holy spirit to move through you to touch the lives of others who have needs.You can also fast to allow the Holy Spirit have is full contral in your life.To allow him guide you.

Acts 10:38 *How God anointed Jesus of Nazareth with the Holy Ghost and with power: who went about doing good, and healing all that were oppressed of the devil; for God was with him*

Isaiah 61:1 *The spirit of the Lord GOD is upon me; because the LORD hath anointed me to preach good tidings unto the meek; he hath sent me to bind up the brokenhearted, to proclaim liberty to the captives, and the opening of the prison to them that are bound;*

Because God has anointed me.

Remember the source of Jesus Christ power was a total link between Him and Heaven

Father you always hear me because I do the things that pleases you" Jon 11:42

This can be said He was in total obedience to God and the word. He did not delay nor did He go ahead of God as time is concerned.

For to everything under the sun there is appointed time.

Ecclesiastes 3:1 *To every thing there is a season, and a time to every purpose under the heaven:*

John 7:*6 To every thing there is a season, and a time to every purpose under the heaven:*

John 2:4 *And they were all filled with the Holy Ghost, and began to speak with other tongues, as the Spirit gave them utterance.*

Acts 1:7-8 *And he said unto them, It is not for you to know the times or the seasons, which the Father hath put in his own power. 8 But ye shall receive power, after that the Holy Ghost is come upon you: and ye shall be witnesses unto me both in Jerusalem, and in all Judaea, and in Samaria, and unto the uttermost part of the earth.*

THE PLACE OF FAITH TO WALK IN MIRACULOUS

Faith flows through revelation of God's word as accompanied

with power

Matt 9:23 *And when Jesus came into the ruler's house, and saw the minstrels and the people making a noise*

Matt 17:21 *Howbeit this kind goeth not out but by prayer and fasting.*

1 Cor 4:20 *For the kingdom of God is not in word, but in power*

Romans 10:8-11*But what saith it? The word is nigh thee, even in thy mouth, and in thy heart: that is, the word of faith, which we preach; 9 That if thou shalt confess with thy mouth the Lord Jesus, and shalt believe in thine heart that God hath raised him from the dead, thou shalt be saved. 10 For with the heart man believeth unto righteousness; and with the mouth confession is made unto salvation. 11 For the scripture saith, Whosoever believeth on him shall not be ashamed.*

Romans 10:17   But what does it say

That if you confess with your mouth the Lord Jesus and believe in your heart that God has raised him From the dead, you will be saved.

For with the heart one believes unto righteousness and with the mouth confession is made unto salvation

For the scripture says "Whoever believes on Him will not be put to shame.

Romans 10:11 **For the scripture saith, Whosoever believeth on him shall not be ashamed**.

So then ....

So we can conclude that when one is on a dry fast, he is not actually starving but feeding as long as you remain hungry for the word of God.

Matt 4:4 ... *But he answered and said, It is written, Man shall not live by bread alone, but by every word that proceedeth out of the mouth of God...............*

The three guiding principle in fasting for anointing and power.

1. It must be led by the Holy spirit and at the appointed

time

Matt 4 :1 ***Then was Jesus led up of the Spirit into the wilderness to be tempted of the devil***

2. It must be a long fast not one day three days or even five days

Matt 4:2 ***And when he had fasted forty days and forty nights, he was afterward an hungered***

Remember with absolute dry fasting one is not go to past 12 days and nights in straight- in a raw.

Use wisdom that God gave you to divide the fasting periods into three or even four .

11 Days and nights in a raw then rest four to seven days take another 11 days and nights then break then you can do the final phase 7 days and nights or even 5 days and nights .

The long fasts should be in three phase per time to avoid putting too much strain on the body .Any fast beyond five days is a long fast .

 If you do shorter fast that do not go beyond five days and nights ,you are free to go even for a year . 5 -5 -5 -5 -5 -5 -5 ....even for a year it is very safe . A doctor put himself on this and cured his cancer .

But remember to start small. You can do 3-5 days and night twice then break for a start to prepare spiritually, physically and psychologically for big one ahead.

That means if you follow strictly the numbers suggested previously you will have fasted between 39 -42 days and nights .

Do not take too long during the breaks, since the power comes gradually but leaves very fast without notice.

To accumulate the power without losing , you need short breaks between the fast that can be between three to five days.

Fasting options .The bold are the fasting days.While the smaller digits are days for refreshment.

45

A) 5-3-7-3-11-3-7- 5-11

b) 3-3-3-3-3-3-3-3-3-3-3-3-3
c) 5-3-5-3-11-5-11-3-7
d) 4-4-4-4-4-4-4-4-4-4-4-4

3. The place of the Word.
Remember during the fast you must cling unto Gods promises. God's Word

You must claim the promises

This is a top secret that will take you to un-imaginable level.

It will bring the fire of the Holy Spirit from heaven.

It will bring the power of the coming world to this present one.

This if done under the influence of the Holy Spirit will change the present day church to the church of latter rain the latter glory- church.

Blind eyes will open with ease

The lunatic/insane /psychotic will become normal with just words of command.

HIV/AIDS will disappear because the power of the blood of Jesus will be too real.

IT will bring one closer to God more quickly than other way known.

This is only for the latter rain revival, anyone else who wants to use it for personal gain God will not allow.

Warning;
If you go with selfish desires the power of God will not be

granted to you. You must go into His presence for His glory for His agenda and His reasons-the right intentions.

Love for God will take you through the love for the lost souls... The urgency to bring them into the fold before it is too late.

The truth on fasting is being revealed to us now that we may secure the greater things of God, that we may receive the gifts of the spirit and that a mighty worldwide revival of spiritual power might sweep over the world with major signs and miracles never seen before.As souls are won to Christ in their millions if not billions . This is the will of God .

If every believer in Christ realize what great power and blessings they are missing without dry fast then they would only be too eager and happy to embrace the Biblical fast and be on the go for Christ.

The in-patients in the national hospital wards need just raw power of God and they will be discharged with just one visiting believer who has fasted the Holy absolute total dry fast for the gifts of healings.

This is mighty but it is not for everyone only the ones God has assigned the duty by the reason of their calling. This power of the Holy Spirit in with the believer is beyond nuclear power in the hands of few scientists.

It can only be done by the one God wants to use for national continental and worldwide revivals.

Because the wisdom of God must be applied to undertake it safely.

Therefore it is not recommended for Tom ,Dick and Hurry believer.

Even though every Christian who is spirit filled can pray and receive mighty power but it must not be mis-used. It is not for sitting at home . You must go out and exercise the power and authority given to you through Christ Jesus.

Do not fast and pray for power of the Holy spirit and then remain idle rather engage in soul winning and exercise the authority of Christ by commanding out the works of satan in people's life. By preaching the gospel of the Kingdom "repent for the kingdom of God is at hand". Matt 4:17

You will be aiming at 40 days and nights dry fast but have to divide according to the time available, wisdom of God and as led by the Holy Spirit. You only need to take one method and stick to the plan.

The place of the word and spirit.

You must be very well equipped with the word. The level of Just like Jesus. The latter rain is coming for the church which has the equal measure of word and spirit. But to do things greater than Jesus did one can still extend the fast beyond 40 days and nights – Just like Moses did two forty days and nights. But this can only be done when you take shorter days of dry fasts and break them frequently or if you do the one so called back to back. The Moses fast. The suggested resting period between two courses of the fast is 30 days .

I mean one can do five days and night dry fast breaking between three to five days. Sixteen times . This will take you a long time between five to seventh months. This needs a very strong will power and determination.

But remember there is one person who did it in the Bible . It is safer and easier

Example

N/B

Bold highlights fasting days while the black one resting and recovery days.

5-3-5-3-5-3-5-**3**-5-3-5-**3**-5-**3**......... forty days maximum

4-3-4-3-4-3-4-3-4-3-4............

5-5-5-5-5-5-5-5-5-5.............

You can go this way even for six years and rest the seventh year(sabbatical laws)

After every six years of work the seventh is for rest. This is for seven times seven then rest for two full years. The sabbatical year and Jubilee.

The year of refreshing , focusing planning , resting, forecasting and reflection. Its time to think.

VERY IMPORTANT: PLAN

Essentially after every long period of intensive fasting you need a good time to recover and rest. You can't be fasting every day.

For an average believer it should be that the recovery periods takes as twice as long as the time you fasted. You cant remain in the mountain forever. You must come down especially for service and your good health.

If you took 21 days and nights to fast then the recovery period should be 42 days and nights before you can undertake another fast.

One can take 11 days and nights to fast that means it should take you 22 days and nights of eating and drinking (recovery) before you can undertake another fast.

But it is also worth noting that under no circumstance should you eat beyond three months without fasting because before you know you will have become carnal Christian.

FASTING AS A LIFESYLE

Dangerous fasting versus right fasting

When you start a fast with wrong intentions for example trying to proove something or fasting in anger ,hatred ,this makes the fasting harmful .

Fasting must be done with the right intentions .You must have no hatred,no unforgiveness in your spirit etc.

Wisdom applies
One week fasting two weeks recovery and rest.
When you have gone into the full spirit it will be one week
fast one week rest.
One month fast one month rest.
This will take time to attain.

Fasting to Heal HIV +

One can break from the jaws of death through long term dry
fasting that reaches between 11-12 days.
1 Cor 15:55
Long term means you can only fast up to 12 days and night
per time then observe the rules of breaking dry fast and if you
are using medicine you continue using your medicine during
recovery period but not during the fasting. Only after breaking the fast. You should resume your medication on the third
day after breaking the fast.
Long terms means you will need 11-12 days and nights dry
fast for more than once, this can take you three or even seven
of them as you continue with your medication and cut off
re- infection sources. Meaning you follow strictly the rules
of not exposing yourself to the virus at all costs. Before you
know you will test negative.
Between the 11 days and nights fast you take 22 days for
recovery. For 12 days and nights fast, you take 24 days and
night recovery before you can fast again.
Long term, may take one year, two or even three years as you
do the 11 or 12 days and nights dry fast.
Remember to claim the healing promises in the scriptures.

Be warned
Dry fasting beyond 12 days and night is fatal. Leads to shut

down of your system and eventually death -clinically . Apply common sense approach. Avoid extremism. Never should you dry fast past 12 days and nights (per time).
It has been proven with clinical cases of people who starve to death especially those in persistance vegetative state ,when all nutrition is denied ,they die from the 12th day and night mark upword . You should never go beyond twelve days and nights per time .

Don't follow your mind – follow knowledge because people perish for lack of knowledge
Hosea 4:6
Don't be led by your determination or frustrations, circumstances or anything else. Acts 27:33-34
And as day was about to dawn Paul implored them all to take food saying " Today is the fourteenth day you have waited and continued without food and eaten nothing. `
Therefore I urge you to take nourishment for this is for your survival.
They were able to do fast for 14 days and nights in an open sea under a great storm. This was a type of soft dry fast .

DRY FASTING IN PREPARATION
FOR RAPTURE GROUND

HolySpirit is the one who will lead the church to the rapture ground after finishing all her assignment here on earth . The church is therfore admonished or instructed not to grieve the Holy Spirit . Bible dry fast will help in putting the flesh down for the HolySpirit to take control and lead .
Everyone preparing for the rapture must be filled with the HolySpirit with the evidence of speaking in tongues .You must be baptised as the early church was in Acts 2:4 .Remember Jesus instructed the early church not to depart from Jeru-

salem until they received the HolySpirit . You must have the HolySpirit just as this disciples in Acts 19:1-9.

A believer would have a sign following -among others speaking in tongues and casting out demons .Mark 16:17 ..You cannot be taken in the rapture if you are not baptised in the HolySpirit with evidence of speaking in tongues . Read Acts 10:45-48.

If you have the blood of Jesus in you heart the next step is to receive the HolySpirit baptism .

How much more will the Heavenly Father give to the Holy-Spirit to them that ask .

Prayer:

Heavenly Father let the blood of your son Jesus Christ wash away all of my sins . In the name of Jesus Christ ,baptism me with the HolySpirit .I receive in Jesus name .Amen

Remember after Elijah had fasted for 40 days and nights and he had some little assignment to take which he did not know about when he was running away from Jezebel and wanted to die .

HE was to anoint Hazael as King over Syria 1 Kings 19:15-16 Jehu as the King of Israel Elisha son of Shapat of Abel Meholah as a prophet in his place.

Elijah did four important things worth noting.

1. He handed over the baton to the right person. Not only did he hand over the baton but he handed it to the right person. Gods choice Elisha 1 Kings 19:16

2. He stopped running away from evil woman instead finished his assignment in grand style – living solution rather than problems behind him. His latter assignment were marked with total clarity and run smoothly

3. He left the mantle of power which is needed on earth not in heaven on the right hands and he also anointed

the right kings.

1 kings 19:15-16

2 Kings 2:13 *He took up also the mantle of Elijah that fell from him, and went back, and stood by the bank of Jordan*

Notice: The mantle was not requested by Elisha nor did Elijah plan to live it but since it was God's perfect will for the demonstration of power to continue on earth. God allowed the mantle to fall off from Elijah, Elisha as led by the spirit picked it and started using it immediately.

4. He went to the rapture ground only with the right person, right attitude and having accomplished Gods mission with His life.

2 kings 2:1 *And it came to pass, when the LORD would take up Elijah into heaven by a whirlwind, that Elijah went with Elisha from Gilgal*

2 Kings 2:11 *And it came to pass, as they still went on, and talked, that, behold, there appeared a chariot of fire, and horses of fire, and parted them both asunder; and Elijah went up by a whirlwind into heaven*

Do you want to be God's friend just like Enoch?

Walking with God until you are no more.

Gen 5:24 *And Enoch walked with God: and he was not; for God took him*

Heb 11:5 *By faith Enoch was translated that he should not see death; and was not found, because God had translated him: for before his translation he had this testimony, that he pleased God*

The end justified the means but more importantly the end of something is better than its beginning

Ecclesistes 7:8 *Better is the end of a thing than the beginning thereof: and the patient in spirit is better than the proud in spirit.*

What legacy do you want to leave behind you?

As a child of God or as a minister of the gospel?

What is this one and only thing you alone could do rather God wants to do through you only and not anybody else?

Why in particular were you born?

Why are you here as such a time as this?

Why did God allow you to even know this secret kept for

ages?

Deuteronomy 29:29*The secret things belong unto the LORD our God: but those things which are revealed belong unto us and to our children for ever, that we may do all the words of this law*.

DRY FASTING FOR FINANCIAL BLESSINGS

Sacrificial giving after dry fasting

You must be a born again Christian, living free from sin.

After giving whole tithe

Giving offering during the services

Helping the poor, knowing that you are lending to God.

Prov 19:17 *He that hath pity upon the poor lendeth unto the LORD; and that which he hath given will he pay him again*

It is important to ask God what He wishes you to offer as a sacrifice – as the Lord but it in your heart.

The perfect sacrifice without blemish is the sacrifice given from the heart which the Lord approves. Without blemish. With total obedience

Just as Abraham heard from God to give his son Isaac as a sacrifice that is the true sacrifice.

Because after giving such a sacrifice all the windows and doors of blessings opens without control

It therefore opens for you.

Blessings that no man can give

Spiritual blessings that lasts beyond your life time .

DRY FASTING FOR LONG LIFE

Only strong viable cells survives a dry fast. Regular fasting are necessary to help restore the protective functions of cells or organs against damage and aging.

The process of fasting improves the mechanism for expelling toxic substances that interfere with body proper functioning ….e .g nitrates pesticides, heavy metals, radio-nuclides and other poisons.

During dry fasting the cells become dehydrated. The dehydrated cells act as furnace burning all sick and weak cells.

Remember dry fasting itself is not a cure but it provides the right conditions to allow the body to activate all of its own God given healing powers and anti aging agents

Those who do regular dry fast live for beyond one hundred years.

Benefits of dry fasting are far reaching.

Tumors can't survive dry fast, fungal infections can't stand dry fast.

What is more?

You need to know all about dry fasting before even attempting one day.

During dry fast you become very sensitive to light, your senses are sharpened and you will be very sensitive to sound. You will be having a burning sensation after some days and nights, it is called the crisis of acidosis. It is more vigorous / very intense with the first timers and the one suffering of a disease. The first crisis of acidosis happens at between day (3-7) then the second and last happens in day nine or ten or even 11th. Remember never to do an absolute dry fast beyond 12th days and nights.

The Pros and Cons

With this Biblical fast you must not eat or drink during the fast.

You must stay where there is proper ventilation – open space or a well ventilated room.

You must not engage in vigorous activities.

You must not do a dry fast when taking a major task e.g exams

You must remain peaceful and joyful avoid things that makes you become angry or overjoyed. Do not get irritated.

Do not bath or wash (avoid any contact with water- by all means)

Should NOT be rained on.

You must plan in advance the dates, day and even onto the hour of starting and breaking the fast.

Do not extend or go beyond the planned (pre-determined) time

Repentance reflection remorse, confession are given the first priorities before asking or knocking the heavens door.

Do not take offence from anyone.

Do not touch dead or come even closer to a corpse than 5 meters.

HEARSAYS ABOUT THE DRY FAST (misunderstandings)

Clearing the misconception.

The false beliefs about Dry fast. The so called myths (hearsays)

1. The major lie about fasting is that without water a person can't survive for over 2-3 days. That the person will dehydrate. Between 50-60 hrs that body start to wither away.

The Truth is

When one stops to eat and drink 400 ml water is formed from a process known as oxidation. This allows fat particles to be broken down forming water. Here are also water stocks in the skin. Scientific studies have shown that from the comfort of a person can't drink or eat for 10 to 12 days.

Therefore all deaths recorded before that time is a result of fear/panic or very extreme condition. Extreme temperature weather hot or cold (weather).

2. Many believe that because there is no special proced-
ure.

During a dry fast that the body will be overburden by the toxins.

But the truth is

That dry fasting deprives body cells of any kind of external power supply, body turns 100% to the inside, allowing cell to do self cleaning.

The body burns more slag and toxins. This causes acceleration of the flow of biochemical reactions accelerating decomposition and oxidation of toxins which increase the bactericidal action of blood 10 times hence it becomes 10 times more dangerous for any harmful microorganism.

At 24-36 hours dry starvation the activity of phagocytes can be increased three times. Autolysis also takes place. It is the process by which the unhealthy and damage tissue are removed from the system.

Autolysis occurs between 2-3 days of dry fasting, but reaching its peak at 8 to 10 days of dry fast. Therefore no enemas needed during dry fast.

3. The third misconception of dry fasting

That dry fasting can cause problems in the kidneys, since they bear a great burden.

But the truth is

When dry fasting the body does not need to recycle water to the extent to which is always done when eating and drinking, however. The kidney and liver are under almost complete rest when dry fasting.

To cause that it is as a result of failure of other organs and system. Kidney does not work alone in the system. It must be remembered that the kidneys are very closely related to the liver.

Most often kidney disease is a consequence of liver failure. Therefore it is very important to do proper cleaning procedures before dry fasting and maintain the right diet after the fast.

When correctly done dry fast cures most of renal diseases and sexually transmitted diseases. It reduces inflammation (swelling).

4. The forth misconception of Dry Fasting

Fasting is a great stress to the body.

But the truth is

Our modern life is full of continuous stress though the worst is that it causes diseases if not dealt with.

Fasting is quite a stress to man just like cold. Though stress itself alone does not mean harm.

When one starves because there is no food is quite different from voluntary fasting.

With psychological preparedness you can dry fast comfortably and get many good results.

It is important to prepare emotionally, mentally and physically. With the right attitude do not force yourself into dry fasting.

5. Misconception Hearsay

That Fasting causes vitamin, Protein and Carbohydrates deficiency

But the Truth is

When fasting the body does not waste energy on digestion, assimilation and separation.

Instead it starts to use nutrients reserves stored in the body.

The stored food not only provides the body with energy bus supply almost all the necessary components for life.

One kilogram of adipose tissue is sufficient for 5 days nutrition.

Dry fasting allows less loss of muscle tissue.

 It breaks the fat tissue since the fat tissues contain 90 % of water.

All the vital organs - heart, brain, and endocrine glands remain intact but much better improve their function.

This is why many who do dry fast end up with creative ability; they become intellectuals – writers, musicians, inventors, renowned artists. They get immeasurably enhanced performance, clearer mind, improved quality of thinking, expansion of influence and associations.

Memory improves in both long term and short term.

6.   The sixth misconception (Hearsay)

That our bodies can by themselves constantly update, so fasting is not necessary. .

But the truth is

Why do we get sick?

Why do we grow old?

Why do we die?

Why do we sometime need some medicine?

If our bodies can constantly update or do the so called auto regulation.

The modern man is oversaturated with poisons of civilization, bad nutrition and unclean environment, therefore his whole life energy is spent in removal of these toxins, this reduces his power to auto regulate.

But with the help of fasting the most natural way man can auto regulate.

Some people look older than their years, others look as their age while others younger and significantly younger than their age.

The human body can easily repair itself, but it needs help to remember how it is done correctly.

7. The Seventh Misconception (Hearsay)

That fasting is ineffective for weight loss

But the truth is :
During fasting extra kilogram quickly go, but just a quick as they went they return if you return to your bad habit of overeating high carbs.
What the Nutritionist say is of course is right. After fasting the body takes full reconstruction process.
 Cells actively absorb nutrients and if at this time you do not limit yourself from bad habits, your weight will quickly return at the same standard and it is likely to exceed its original by several kilos.
Therefore the goal of the fasting must not only be to lose weight but to completely change behaviors. (Bad eating habits- which includes overeating and eating junk food) that brought you obesity
Blood pressure drops to normal
Shortness of breath disappears
Heart tones became normal
Women restore the correct menstrual cycle
Men restore potency
People with mental disorder returns to normal
It is harmless no side effect.

The easiest and best way to lose weight with dry fast is to do alternate day fast .Fast one day rest one day.

During Fasting

There is a fast and safe loss of weight.
Man tolerates hunger easily there are no hunger pangs.
There are no sagged over flabby skin or tissue s
Weight loss during fasting is accompanied by rehabilitation of the body and improving overall health.
Fasting helps to fight bad eating habits.
For one to overcome obesity it is necessary to do combination of the fasting.
Both dry and water fast, several of them in a raw.

Change your diet to lacto – vegetarian. Thoroughly chew food- (carefully chew food before swallowing.

Then to weekly fast.

Reduce amount of food on each of your plate. Change the size of your plate to smaller ones.

8. The eighth misconception – (Hearsay)

Many people who believe in dry fasting claim that dry fasting can cure any incurable diseases and even cancer in the fourth stage.

But the truth is

Dry fast cannot heal broken bones, but can cause the swelling and inflammation of water to disappear as quickly as possible. Prolonged dry fasting is very effective in severe disease as rheumatoid, arthritis, ankylosing, spondylitis. Arthrosis deformans etc.

It absorbs ovarian cysts.

It makes benign tumors to disappear.

But as a drowning man will clutch at a straw many run to dry fasting when it is too late, when all natural defenses in the body are completely destroyed and the sick is hopeless – then they start the fast without preparation – prior purification or raining of the body. This results to serious complications and the outcome is death. .

Cancer can be cured through dry fast but at the initial stage, by taking few courses of dry fasting, leaving the city life and going to natural clean environment. Preferably forested area.

To live in nature, completely change your lifestyle whenever you are then you can be sure of good results.

Most importantly all things need to be done on time before it is too late. (A stitch in time saves nine)

During fasting of course some may die but it is not because of the fasting but because of the fact that the body is overfed to failure with all sorts of filth.

A terminally ill man may die during fasting not because of

the fast but as a result of the illness/disease.

For example people have died for their own ignorance, by not observing the laws that guides on breaking fasting.

N/B

This is not death as a result of fasting but of exiting from fasting by eating heavy meals to break a long fast. Is Foolishness at its best and fatal at its worst.

9. The ninth misconception (Hearsay)

Many people write that during the dry fasting one should do enema of salt water and rinse the mouth with water. It helps to go through the fasting easier.

But the truth is

During dry fasting the cells of our bodies begin to develop its own high quality water from its own internal reserves and therefore in contact with water in the mouth or intestine this process (mechanisms) is broken.

It only provokes thirst which makes the passage continuing dry fast impossible.

Leading to breaking fast prematurely.

Go gain your health you have to work and work with patience through long suffering – which leads to cleaning and purification which is the greatest goal of man.

ADVANTAGES OF DRY FAST

Dry fasting has a lot of advantages over all the other types of fasting.

Researchers have proved it that for a completely healthy rat it takes 12 days and nights of dry fast to die.

In the wilderness when animals get sick they stop drinking and eating for a number of consecutive days before they resume.

One of the most feared weapon of war is nuclear bomb .Dry fasting for 5 days and nights enables you to have immunity against all radiation effects-before the exposure. But if incase you exposed yourself you need only seven days and nights to cure radiation effects.Dry fast is that powerful .

Super benefits of dry fasting.

i)   Deep refreshment and calmness within (no worries, fear, panic, stress, the noise within is silenced.|)

ii)   Increase in reception ability

iii)   Increase tactile, skin sensitivity(smooth and smart skin)

iv)   Enhances sense of smell

v)   Enhances sense of touch

vi)   Awakens the healing energy in the body.

vii)   It opens ability to understand people without words (telepathic abilities)

viii)   Helps to develop strong will power if done as life-style. Regular fasting

ix)   Remember we need unshakable determination to have good success in every life endeavors.

x)   Makes one to have understanding and compassion for the hungry and the poor since you too experience what they pass through.

xi)   Helps one to be sensitive on what amounts of water and food the body need. You no longer overeat or drink. But take only reasonable and necessary amount of food and drink as per the body requirement.

xii)   After dry fasting your skin develops good proper resistance against cold

xiii)   Gray hair turns thicker and younger in colour

xiv)   Improves the sense of sight.

xv)   Makes yellow eyeball turn pure white

xvi)   IF you were snoring in you sleep after dry fast, breathing become smooth and quiet.

xvii)   Gnashing of teeth stops

xviii) If you have had a heavy breath, the breath become clear and you develop a clear and bad breath disappear.

xix)   It makes sensation in the sweet and fresh especially if you had problems with bitter mouth in the morning.

xx)   The yellow plague on the teeth turns white as pearls.

xxi)   If your teeth were loosely attached the gums after dry fast the gums become stronger therefore a firm tight teeth.

xxii)   Chronic running nose is cured completely.

xxiii)   Dry fast brings back pressure to normal.

xxiv)   After dry fast there is increase in strength hence superb potency.

xxv)   A healthy man or woman looks younger after a dry fast 10-15 years younger.

xxvi)   Dry fasting helps to maximize development of the sensory perception - it opens one to spiritual world allowing vision, spiritual gifts, flow of heavenly wisdom.

xxvii)   It allows for self- fulfillment and achievement of harmony for the whole person, body soul and spirit.

What to do during the process of dry fasting.

Breath through the nose avoids breathing through the mouth.

Early in the morning make three deep breath of fresh air and repeat the same late in the evening.

Feel your mind with the word of God. Meditate upon the word of God. Eliminate every negative thought and emotions.

Help people that you can, especially the sick, hurting, and needy and do it with Joy.

Repent over greed, laziness, fear, hypocrisy, pride, complacency all form of evil.

Believe people and love them.

Do not talk about anyone unfairly

Do not take close to your heart unkind opinions about people.

Liberate your mind from thinking about diseases, pain, ailments, demons, and even death. This is the secret of victory.

Believe in God and His power. For with God all things are possible.

Accept the fact that all human needs can be met including yours through Gods word. Keep searching the scriptures and revelation (deeper understanding)

Tell yourself today and only today I am a hero/heroine not tomorrow to avoid postponing the fast.

How to breakfast safely

For a number of days treat your stomach as that of a new born baby and vice versa.

Treat your stomach as that of a young baby for a number of days.

Take water in sips and rolling it in your mouth before swallowing. You must take at least 2 litres of water in a period of 2 hours. Everything must be done in order without hurrying

After the two hours you can now take yogurt or ice cream milk (mala)

Slowly return to animal protein mostly in liquid form. (soup and broth)

Mashed potatoes

Noodles (indomie , spaghetti)

Drink much clean water as possible

You must time yourself that is from when to when. (Sunset to sunset)

Take shower bath.

After 12 hours you must have a warm protein broth(soup)

Gradually feed yourself with the very soft protein (fish)

Cooked vegetables

Use very little salt in your food in the early days after breaking the fast.

Avoid canned foods

Avoid processed foods and saturated sugar products

Remember exit from dry fasting must be strictly observed because it is more important than the process of fasting itself.

After fasting the body is very clean, so you can only feed it with very clean fresh, highly quality products.

Avoid exposure to cold or too much sunshine

IF you are in an area where there is less humidity- limit yourself to shorter dry fasts .

Mandatory rule as of Dry Fasting (Must be followed.)

Rule one

Breaking of a long dry Fast (Long duration of fasting Dry takes two or more days)

After the dry fast the body becomes pure so it should be reloaded only with clean, fresh, high quality products with no germs-dirt's or disease causing micro-organism.

Break of Dry Fast Must be strict because the breaking of dry fast is more important than the process of the dry fast.

If the beginning of the dry fast occurred for example at 19:00 hours the last water was consumed then the break of dry fast should also happen at 19:00 hours (even 5 minutes before is not allowed).

N/B In the case of 36 hour Dry Fast. If the fast commenced at 19:00 hours then it will end at 7:00 o'clock in the morning the day after.

At 19:00 hours you can brush your teeth and drink cool (especially chilled) clean, boiled water – as much as you want, you can use a lemon. It should be drunk in small doses with breaks during the first two hours.

It is not allowed to drink warm, hot or mineral or raw (unprocessed) spring, nor any other water.

Unprocessed spring water means water straight from the natural resources.

In very rare cases, the first sips of water might ease nausea, and then every sip of water should be kept in the mouth, mixing it with saliva and then swallowing in about 20-30 seconds. As you drink water you can also take shower,. After showering it's good to pour over yourself some cold water, and then take a warm bath.

It should not take more than 8 minutes. Along with washing continue drinking water till 21:00 hours (for the next two hours)

At 21:00 hours consume animal protein in the form of milk products. Yogurt as much desired, in small portions.

It is allowed to eat organic or homemade cottage cheese, while consuming it is no feeling of heaviness in the stomach.

At 23:00 hours eat a warm protein based broth (as much as desired), fish or chicken no vegetables, well cooked no salt and no bread.

The soup can be cooked with spices (but do not eat the spices).

After the dry fast eating should be resumed with small portions. This extended fast breaking time is necessary for gradually increasing load on the pancreases which has been dormant during the fasting and should now be carefully re-engaged back to its work.

Rule two for the first two days

The first two days after dry fast must include drinking of

pure water, eating mainly fresh protein – rich foods of animal's origin. Fatty yogurt, cottage cheese, sour cream, cheese, fish and chicken broth boiled fish, chicken, eggs etc

On the second day in the morning you can eat slice of bread (no yeast is better) and in the evening hot cereal(oatmeal) or boiled vegetables.

Within the first 2 days you cannot eat raw vegetables and fruits, and raw foods of plants origin.

IF you have eaten something wrong and you feel nauseous, or you experience a metallic taste in the mouth or have a rotten egg tasting burps or swelling appeared you must urgently drink a glass or two or three of ice-cream milk (mala) and switch back to animal protein.

Rule 2 is mandatory for everyone including vegetarian. This does not contradict a vegetarian diet. This is necessary because after the dry Fast, body is in a dire need of "building material "that is animal protein for the synthesis of proteins and new cells.

Violation of rule 2 can lead to negative consequences.

IF you do not consume meat or sea food and dairy, pick the most protein rich plants, fruits and veggies for your recovery period.

Starting from the third day you can resume foods that are well cooked.

That is

Fish, poultry, eggs, any dairy products, honey, fruits dried fruit, berries, raw and cooked vegetables, mushrooms, nuts, seaweeds, wheat bran, various hot cereals, soaked seeds of grains and legumes.

Allowed to drink: clean filtered water, no-sugar added juices herbal tea, mineral water.

You should also take food rich in calcium that is well cooked fish head and bones, honey. The food should be diverse and well saturated with vitamin and micro-macro elements.

During the first five days after the break of dry fast use only fresh, clean and high quality products.

You cannot eat salt

Salt Containing foods

Sugar

Sugar products

During this period beware of infection nitrates, diseases causing microorganism etc

RULE THREE

During the complete period of dry fasting especially in days of fasting it is necessary to air the room, often perform; breathing exercises body needs a periodic light physical activities and oxygen

RULE FOUR

Under no circumstances should the predetermined length of fast be extended since it corresponds to a pre programmed psychological state.

For example, if you prepare for four days fast it is not allowed to move to five days fast even in every good health condition. Consequently, if you are not tolerating hunger well, you can always break ahead of time, observing the rules of strict breaking of dry fasting.

Rule FIVE

For the first time dry fasting is allowed only with one day fasting, moving gradually to two, three four and then five.

RULE SIX

During the dry fast it is not allowed to use any drugs, do not relief the pain and tolerate it instead. If the pain is unbearable, then you can break the fast ahead of time, observing the rules of strict fast breaking.

RULE SEVEN

Before fasting, during fasting and after fasting no enemas are needed, since the absorption of toxin from the gastro-intestinal tract is absent due to lack of water.

Comments

On the crisis of acidosis

The regeneration process may occur with strong pain, and one should be prepared for that. In the initial stages of dry fast crisis of acidosis can happen on the fifth day in the future on the 4th, 3rd or even 2nd day after starting dry fast.

The sooner the crisis comes, the faster it passes, the more time remains to renew the body.

Self dry fasting a very serious business. Everyone is responsible for themselves.

CONDITIONS FOR OBTAINING POSITIVE RESULTS

Have faith in the benefits of dry fast

Meditate on the word of God .

Healthy lifestyle

Confidence in the existence of large reserve capacity of your own body

Strict adherence to the chosen method of dry fast.

Loving all and having a good mood .

Hard work on mind development, because only the higher level of consciousness is able to create and maintain a high level of the physical body.

USEFUL INFORMATION FOR DRY FAST

Dry fast is tolerated much more easily than water fasting and juice. The first dry fast (most difficult) should be fractionated / divided

It is helpful to make a calendar schedule for the total period of dry fast including days of the week.

It is best to plan a break of dry fast for the weekend.

It is important to plan a menu for in between days of fasting.

It is necessary to prepare and stock up in advance yogurt, broth and other products with possible early exit from the dry fast.

Purification of the person fasting occurs not only during the dry fasting but also after.

Develop friendly relationship for consultation with people who have experience in dry fasting

During Dry fasting do not take offence from anyone (do not be angry at anyone)

Be kind to everyone

Do not get irritated

Do not argue

Do not scold

Do not allow negative emotions (avoid negativity even in thoughts and words)

Notice there is a big difference between five one day dry fast (break every evening) and a complete five days and nights dry fast (continuous).

During the fast one should save the body strength and not waste any energy.

The number of eating days between the fasts can be increased at personal discretion/ choice in order to gain weight for subsequent period of fasting. It is advisable to conduct the 24-or 36 hour dry fast weekly

Five days dry fast after every three months

Clearly put in your mind the breaking time when you start (open) a dry fast.

Do not be fooled by pleasant feeling of lightness and health after the dry fast. IF you are not planning to change your body life and raise your spiritual level, your body after some time will return to its former state. The process of dry fast is sometimes different for everyone because it depends on the environmental factors and the individuals.

Fasting longer for 9,10, 11,or 12 days should be done in nature new clean rivers, or in the woods. Where the environment is clean away from polluted water or air.

MY OWN EXPERIENCE
AND TESTIMONIES

The first time I dry fasted I was scared to death,used to go to the mirrow and check my eye balls.If it was red that meant the fast was working against me so I discontinued.I had fasted 14 days with juices then three days water fast.I dry fasted forty eight hours the first time then because there was something red in one of my eyes I stopped.I had not done proper detox that is why I had the redness in the corner of my eye.Then I dry fasted again another 3 days and nights but this time round I reached the acidosis crisis,there was a burning in my body like fire.After I broke the fast I felt very light in in my body.I did another forty eight hours.I did another and another so many I lost the count .During this series of the fast I asked the Lord for the gift of word of knowledge and to confirm that I had received the Lord physically sent a light which rested on my chest.I would walk with it wherever I went within my place of residence not public.At night it was resting on the top of the bed.I heard never seen anything like that.Then it started to operate.Before a person could come to visit me I would know even the purpose of the visit before they arrived.If you talked to me and there was something you are hiding or you don't know I would know.I used to have dreams on the events that were yet to happen,but after getting this gift those dreams became very accurate.While in the dream it looks so real that I remember every detail when am awake .

 In another event a thief broke into my house stole the valuable which included all my electronics.My friend ,I got into dry fast,five days and nights and rested,then after three days fasted again another five days,then another.Just after the series of the fasts he was caught.The power of the Holy Spirit worked so dramatic ,where he went to hide after he was found out-he felt drowsy and could no longer run .Just like that he was caught and he returned all the things he had stollen .
One of my friend after doing a series of about two days ,his life just improved he had to migrate.
Another of my friends, I fasted for them to get a baby.Another of my friends fasted five days and night only and got a new job and did a glorious wedding.Another friend of mine we fasted together-co-operate fasts and got a well paying job and later wedded.

My wife got a healing miricle of tumor in the breast after series of dry fast one reaching eight days and another six days.Dry fast has instant miraclous results,whether be it financial issues,health issues,spiritual issues.We don't always fast ourselves to death to get the results,just a little fast with persistance produce results.
I know of a man who wanted to leave his wife and children to get married to another lady .The common marital issues but the wife had just learnt about dry fast and she fasted upto eight days and night and that was the end of the problem .They lived happy ever after .

I learnt about dry fasting directly through the Holy Spirit. One time I was walking the streets of Nairobi to be precise Harambee Avenue while undertaking water fast. I went to buy mineral water and suddenly the Holy Spirit held my hands before I could pay for the water(stop I want to show you a better and excellent way")

And He called it "HEBREW FAST" From that time I started to research until I got all the information necessary including the Biblical examples
I straight away embrace the fasting and started immediately.
Though in the initial stages after breaking the fast always had problems with eating heavy ugali (cooked flour in hot water)
But later after learning the laws of breaking the fast and observing them to the latter I did not have problems again with the stomach.
Fungal infections disappeared
Oppression by demons spirits stopped
One time a very bright light landed on my own chest over my

sweater.

I started to understand the scriptures very deeply and differ-ently.

Every habit that made my Christian questionable just vanished.

I felt lighter in my body and very sober/alert in the mind .

I cried oh how comes I did not know this from the beginning of my faith walk .

I had practiced juice fasting for over ten years and even water fast but the power of dry fast was quite strong and different so I ceased the juice and water fasting.

During the dry fasting whatever I ask in prayer I always get imme-diately response from heaven.

The Holy Spirit voice became very clear.

I see clear dreams no guesswork.

FASTING HELPS IN PERSECUTION

Mathews 10: 23 *But when they persecute you in this city, flee ye into an-other: for verily I say unto you, Ye shall not have gone over the cities of Israel, till the Son of man be come.*

BROTHER YUN (1995)

A Chinese born preacher an evangelist brother Yun has both suffered incredibly hardship and experienced the most amazing of miracles.

Refusing to join the official Christian Church of China he was im-prisoned and tortured in the notorious Zhengzhou maximum Se-curity Prison. During this time Bro. Yun claims to have engaged in a total 75 days fasting He was the only person ever to escape Zhengzhou Prison. Brother Yun also claims to have been granted the power of invisibility to escape his oppressors.

CONCLUSION

Those who do frequent fasts ,their body get used to the state and this help them fast easily without so many preparation .But it is important to have a very clean gut without anything in the intestine before you start a long dry fast .

 Water fast is only to help you do a dry fast .

Fasting without water and food beyond five days at home is not recommend in this book.It is only suggested .Though many are now doing it at home safely ,listening to your body is the secret.

At home you can safely fast up to a maximum of 5 days and rights in a raw. I do upto six days at home safely .

If you have to go beyond 5 days and rights you need close supervision, experienced dry faster and it must be done in clean environment away in the nature if possible. . . .

Your victory comes through Jesus Christ the Holy Spirit and God the father through His word and spirit.

You need to confess victory during and even after the fast even if you are not seeing any. Victory always comes after the fast.

Have faith in what you have done and learnt to hand over your case to God. Closing the chapter behind and focusing ahead. Let the weak say " I am strong " Joel 3:10

I can do all things through Christ Jesus who strengthens me. Philipians 4:13

Remember the wild animals in the wild only follow their instincts no book to read , no ambulance for emergency cases, no diagnosis yet when sick they dry fast and break safely.

Let's learn from the nature to follow our instincts. Meet you in New Jerusalem.

BE BORN AGAIN

God did not ask Adam if he wanted to be created. None of us were asked if we want to be born but we are asked if we want 1 *And it came to pass, when men began to multiply on the face of the earth, and daughters were born unto them, 2 That the sons of God saw the daughters of men that they were fair; and they took them wives of all which they chose.*

3 And the LORD said, My spirit shall not always strive with man, for that he also is flesh: yet his days shall be an hundred and twenty years.

4 There were giants in the earth in those days; and also after that, when the sons of God came in unto the daughters of men, and they bare children to them, the same became mighty men which were of old, men of renown. 5 And God saw that the wickedness of man was great in the earth, and that every imagination of the thoughts of his heart was only evil continually.

6 And it repented the LORD that he had made man on the earth, and it grieved him at his heart.   7 And the LORD said, I will destroy man whom I have created from the face of the earth; both man, and beast, and the creeping thing, and the fowls of the air; for it repenteth me that I have made them.

8 But Noah found grace in the eyes of the LORD.   9 These are the generations of Noah: Noah was a just man and perfect in his generations, and Noah walked with God

To be born again

When Noah built the ark (Gen 6:1-9)

He had local helpers whom he possibly paid. They may have accepted the money but not the invitation to enter and perished. Only the eight members of Noah's family entered and were saved. Yes it is possible to help build Gods Kingdom today, but never enter it.

A sobering thought. The hand of God finally locked the door. The same hand that locked Noah and his family in locked the rest of the people OUT.

Do not be deceived, God is not mocked (Gal 6:7) *Be not deceived; God is not mocked: for whatsoever a man soweth, that shall he also reap*

IF you unsaved or a back slider and not ready for Heaven today, say the sinners' prayer right now:

Ooh God save my soul! I am so sorry I have sinned against you. But I have come home. I may have doubted your love, your truth and your grace many times, but forgive me, LORD. You said if you I would repent and be as sorry for my sins as God is that I committed them, you would forgive me and save me through the divine blood. I am sorry and I do confess my sins and I believe the blood of Jesus washes them all away right now. Come into my heart, Jesus! Come on in!

If you meant that prayer, He is yours and now you can say Hallelujah, Jesus is mine.

Healing prayer:

Lord Jesus Christ ,heal me from all the diseases in my body .
Heal ,heal ,heal .